# COMPLETE GUIDE TO

# GANGRENE

# AMPUTATION

Comprehensive Handbook To Diagnosis, Prevention, Treatment, And Recovery Strategies For Optimal Health Outcomes

## DR. BRUNO HORAN

# Disclaimer:

The information provided in this book, is intended for general informational purposes only and should not be considered as professional advice.

The author has made every effort to ensure the accuracy of the information presented. However, readers are advised to consult with a qualified healthcare professional before attempting any herbal remedies or making significant changes to their wellness routine. Individual health conditions vary, and what may be suitable for one person may not be appropriate for another.

It is important to note that the author is not in any endorsement deal, partnership, or affiliation with any organization, brand, or company mentioned in this book. Any references to specific products or services are based on the author's personal experience or general knowledge and do not imply an endorsement or promotion of those products or services

## Contents

# CONCERNING THIS BOOK

"Gangrene Amputation" is a vital resource that explores the intricate and frequently upsetting circumstances surrounding gangrene as well as the crucial decision-making process involved in amputation. This book serves as a thorough reference that has been painstakingly arranged to cover every aspect of various medical issues. It offers priceless insights for patients, caregivers, and medical professionals alike.

The first few chapters provide a general overview of gangrene, including information on its different forms, including gas, wet, dry, and Fournier's gangrene. Readers obtain a more complex understanding of the genesis of this ailment by delving into the core reasons, which include infections, long-term illnesses, and trauma. Detailed descriptions of symptoms such as discoloration, swelling, and bad odor are essential for prompt diagnosis and treatment. Additionally, the thorough explanation of diagnosis, which includes physical examinations, imaging, and laboratory tests, gives readers the information they need to recognize gangrene quickly and accurately and emphasizes the value of receiving treatment as soon as possible.

The serious repercussions of untreated gangrene are brought to light by complications including sepsis and the spread of infection to adjacent tissues. This prepares us for the next important subject: amputation. The book presents a thorough analysis of the many amputation methods, making a distinction between surgeries involving the lower and upper limbs, and presents a fair assessment of the benefits and drawbacks of each kind. A personal touch is added by case studies and patient narratives, which highlight the practical consequences and results of various medical choices.

Another major focus of this book is surgical preparation, which includes everything from psychological counseling and family support to medical examinations and tests. It highlights the all-encompassing strategy required for excellent surgical results, along with what to anticipate on the day of operation, which helps to allay patient fears and guarantee they are prepared and aware.

An extensive examination of the methods and procedures used in amputation surgery can be found under the section on surgical procedures. It gives patients a clear understanding of what to expect by going over anesthetic and pain management, the length of the procedure, and immediate post-operative care. In-depth examinations of wound care, pain management techniques, post-surgical recovery, and the vital role of physical therapy and rehabilitation guarantee that readers comprehend the entire treatment needed for recovery.

Prosthetics and rehabilitation are covered extensively, including the kinds of prosthetics, fitting and customizing them, and the physical therapy required to use them. Testimonials and success stories from people who have had amputations provide hope and inspiration by demonstrating the potential for recovery of independence and quality of life.

The prevention of problems, regular medical check-ups, and required lifestyle modifications are all important aspects of long-term care and management. The resources and support groups that offer patients and their families a network of both practical and emotional help are highlighted.

A comprehensive examination of living with an amputation is provided, along with tools and procedures for everyday living as well as methods for preserving independence. A major emphasis is on overcoming social and emotional obstacles, and there are motivational anecdotes that highlight the tenacity and accomplishments of those who have had amputations.

The most recent developments in prosthetics and surgical methods are covered in advanced themes and future directions, highlighting the continuous advancements in this discipline. An essential resource for understanding these intricate medical journeys, the book also discusses research and clinical trials, the role of technology in rehabilitation, and the outlook for gangrene therapy and amputation in the future.

# CHAPTER ONE

## COMMUNICATION WITH GANGRENE

A dangerous illness known as gangrene develops when a substantial portion of body tissue perishes from a lack of blood supply.

There are several causes for this, such as wounds, infections, and long-term illnesses. Tissues that are deprived of oxygen and nutrients due to a reduction in blood flow eventually deteriorate and die. If gangrene is not treated right away, it can result in potentially fatal consequences and is frequently accompanied by excruciating pain, discoloration, and an unpleasant smell.

## Fournier's, Wet, Gas, And Dry Gangrene Types

There are multiple forms of gangrene, each with unique traits and underlying causes:

Dry gangrene: This kind is usually brought on by a persistent reduction in blood supply to a specific region, frequently as a result of diseases like diabetes or atherosclerosis. The afflicted tissue turns dark brown or black, shrivels up, and becomes dry. Generally speaking, it advances more slowly and is less prone to become infected than other forms of gangrene.

Wet Gangrene: A bacterial infection is the cause of wet gangrene, as opposed to dry gangrene. The affected area looks wet and shiny, gets bloated, and develops blisters. It spreads quickly and is accompanied by an odorous discharge. To stop additional tissue damage and consequences, wet gangrene needs to be treated medically immediately.

Gas Gangrene: The bacteria Clostridium perfringens, which creates gas and toxins within the afflicted tissues, is the cause of this severe form of gangrene. Gas gangrene is marked by excruciating agony, swelling, and the appearance of gas bubbles beneath the skin. It advances very quickly, frequently within hours. It's a medical emergency that needs to be attended to right away.

Fournier's Gangrene: The vaginal and perineal areas are the only areas affected by this kind. This rare but potentially fatal form of necrotizing fasciitis occurs when bacteria enter the soft tissues and quickly kill the tissue. Aggressive antibiotic therapy and timely surgical intervention are necessary for Fournier's gangrene.

## Causes: Chronic Illnesses, Injuries, And Infections

Gangrene can occur due to several factors:

Infections: Clostridium species infections in particular can quickly demolish tissues and result in gangrene. Wounds and surgical sites are frequently the sites of these infections.

Chronic Diseases: Atherosclerosis, diabetes, and peripheral artery disease can all reduce blood flow, which increases the risk of gangrene in tissues. Diabetes patients with poorly managed blood sugar levels might damage blood vessels, which reduces circulation.

Accidents: Serious wounds like burns, frostbite, or crush injuries can stop blood flow to the area that is injured, which raises the possibility of gangrene. Treatment delays and inadequate wound care can increase this risk.

Symptoms: Swelling, Odor, Discoloration

Gangrene manifests in a variety of ways that can notify people of its existence:

Discoloration: As the tissue dies, the affected area may first appear red before changing to brown, black, or green. This discoloration frequently serves as a crucial gangrene warning.

Swelling: Blisters and skin swelling are common, especially in cases of gas and wet gangrene. The area may also feel painful and heated to the touch.

Foul Odor: Gangrene is frequently accompanied by a distinct, foul-smelling discharge, particularly in cases of wet and gas gangrene. The decay of dead tissue and the presence of bacterial infection cause the stench.

## Diagnosis: Lab Tests, Imaging, And Physical Exam

To properly diagnose gangrene and determine its severity, several actions must be taken:

Physical Exam: The first stage is a comprehensive physical examination by a medical professional. In addition to looking for indications of infection, they will evaluate the affected area's look, color, and temperature.

Imaging: Methods like MRIs, CT scans, and X-rays can be used to assess the amount of tissue damage and identify any gas in the tissues, which is a sign of gas gangrene.

Lab testing: To determine the precise bacteria causing the infection and to assess the patient's general health, laboratory testing such as tissue cultures and blood tests are crucial. Blood testing can also detect indicators of sepsis, a severe systemic illness.

## Sepsis And Spread To Other Tissues Are Complications

If gangrene is not treated right away, it can cause major complications:

Sepsis: One of the most dangerous side effects of gangrene is sepsis, a potentially fatal illness in which the body's reaction to an infection results in extensive inflammation. If left untreated, sepsis can result in organ failure and even death.

Spread to Other Tissues: If gangrene is not treated, it may spread to surrounding muscles and tissues, exacerbating the condition and raising the possibility of amputation. Additionally, the infection can spread via the blood, leading to systemic problems.

Preventing serious consequences and guaranteeing improved health results require an understanding of the intricacies of gangrene, the ability to identify its symptoms, and prompt medical care.

# CHAPTER TWO

## CATEGORIES OF AMPLIFIERS

### Lower Limb Amputations

Amputating a toe

The removal of one or more toes owing to gangrene is known as a toe amputation. When alternative therapies fail to control localized gangrene, this kind of amputation is frequently required. The process is not too complicated and can stop the virus from spreading. But losing a toe might change one's gait and balance, necessitating certain walking adjustments.

Amputation of the Foot

A foot amputation is the removal of a section of the foot, which may include the midfoot, the forefoot, or one or more toes. When gangrene is still contained within the foot but has progressed past the toes, this kind of amputation is usually carried out. For patients receiving this treatment to regain mobility and adjust to alterations in their gait, prosthetic devices and therapy may be necessary.

Amputation Below the Knee

In a below-knee amputation (BKA), the leg is amputated below the knee. When gangrene affects the lower leg but is contained below the knee, this surgery is required. BKA protects the knee joint, which is essential for preserving the range of motion and enhancing the patient's capacity to use a prosthetic limb.

Amputation Above the Knee

The process of above-knee amputation (AKA) entails amputating the leg above the knee. If the gangrene has spread above the knee, this is necessary. Even while AKA causes a greater loss of function than BKA, patients can still acquire a high level of mobility and independence because of developments in prosthetic technology and rehabilitation methods.

## Amputations Of The Upper Limbs

Amputation of Fingers

A finger amputation is the removal of a finger or fingers because of gangrene. The function of the hand can be severely impacted by this kind of amputation, particularly if numerous fingers are lost. However, patients can frequently learn how to carry out daily duties efficiently with the use of adaptive technology and physical therapy.

Amputation of the Hand

A hand amputation is the removal of all or a portion of the hand. This treatment is carried out when the hand is severely affected by gangrene. Because hands are essential for daily activities and fine motor abilities, losing one can be especially difficult. Adaptive techniques and prosthetic hands can help restore some function.

Amputation Below the Elbow

An arm is amputated below the elbow joint in a procedure known as below-elbow amputation (BEA). When gangrene is present in the forearm but can be contained below the elbow, this surgery is chosen. Greater functional potential with a prosthetic limb is made possible by BEA, which maintains the elbow joint.

Amputation Above the Elbow

Amputation above the elbow (AEA) is the removal of the arm above the elbow joint. If the gangrene has progressed past the elbow, this is required. Although AEA can have a major influence on functionality and range of motion, patients can adapt and regain independence with the aid of contemporary prosthetics and rehabilitation programs.

Gangrene's severity and extent

The degree and scope of the gangrene are the main factors determining the kind of amputation. In cases where gangrene is limited, a little amputation, like removing a finger or toe, may be sufficient. To make sure the infection is completely eradicated, more severe cases of gangrene can require a larger degree of amputation.

The general health of the patient

The kind and extent of amputation depends on the patient's overall health, including the existence of diseases like diabetes or peripheral artery disease. individuals with more health issues might need less invasive surgeries, while healthier individuals might recover better from more thorough amputations.

The Vascular Supply

The vitality of the blood supply to the injured limb is an important factor. Higher levels of amputation may be necessary in cases with poor vascular supply to guarantee adequate blood flow and good healing of the remaining limb.

Practical Aspects

Another important consideration is the possible effect on the patient's function and mobility. Aiming to maintain as much limb function as feasible, surgeons consider how the patient's ability to use prosthetic devices and perform daily activities will be impacted by the amputation.

## Pros And Cons Of Every Category

Amputating a toe

Benefits: Less invasive, quicker recuperation, and decreased chance of issues. Cons: If gangrene spreads, there may be a risk of more amputations and impairments to gait and balance.

## Amputation of the Foot

Advantages: Preserves portion of the leg for movement and removes more extensive gangrene. Cons: Rehab and prosthetics are required, and walking and balance are significantly impacted.

## Amputation Below the Knee

Advantages: Less complications than higher amputations, better mobility with prosthesis, preservation of the knee joint. Cons: Major surgery, prolonged rehabilitation, and prosthesis adaptation.

## Amputation Above the Knee

Advantages: Better results are possible with prostheses, which are essential for severe gangrene patients. Cons: Requires considerable rehabilitation; increases energy consumption during walking; results in greater loss of mobility.

## Amputation of Fingers

Positives: Faster recuperation and less impact than in the case of higher limb amputations. Cons: May influence quality of life and impair hand function and dexterity.

Amputation of the Hand

Advantages: Eliminates severe gangrene; may lead to useful prosthesis. Cons: Profound loss of function, difficulties carrying out daily duties, and requirement for significant adjustments.

Amputation Below the Elbow

Advantages: Better chance of using a prosthetic functionally, preserves elbow joint. Cons: Requires extensive rehabilitation; affects arm function; requires major surgery.

Amputation Above the Elbow

Advantages: Eliminates widespread gangrene; may lead to more sophisticated prosthesis. Cons:

Significant loss of range of motion and function; extensive adaption is needed.

## Patient Narratives And Case Studies

Case Study: John's Amputation Below the Knee

John, a diabetic patient who was sixty-two years old, had lower limb gangrene. The gangrene worsened despite early treatments, requiring amputation below the knee.

John went through a rigorous rehabilitation program after surgery to learn how to operate a prosthetic leg. He experienced a marked improvement in his quality of life, regained his mobility, and resumed his favorite activities within six months.

Patient Narrative: Amputation of Mary's Finger

Due to a serious infection, Mary, a 45-year-old office worker, developed gangrene in her index finger. Following her amputation of a finger, Mary first had difficulty doing everyday duties. She adjusted gradually with the aid of adaptive equipment and occupational therapy. Mary has resumed her work with little difficulty and now employs assistance aids, demonstrating her adaptability and perseverance.

Case Study: Tom's Amputation Above the Elbow

Tom, a thirty-year-old mechanic, broke his forearm due to a severe injury. To preserve his life, an amputation was done above the elbow.

Tom had a difficult rehabilitation, but he was able to learn how to operate a cutting-edge prosthetic limb with the help of a multidisciplinary team.

Tom now takes part in local activities and has discovered new passions, proving the value of all-encompassing rehabilitation.

Patient Narration: Lisa's Amputated Foot

Due to gangrene, Lisa, a 55-year-old woman with peripheral artery disease, had to have her foot amputated. Following her operation, Lisa had severe trouble balancing and walking.

She adjusted to her new situation with tenacious rehabilitation and the usage of bespoke orthotics. Lisa currently helps out at an amputee support group, where she encourages and supports people going through similar struggles.

# CHAPTER THREE

## GETTING READY FOR SURGERY

A thorough plan must be followed to ensure both physical and mental preparedness for gangrene amputation surgery.

Comprehensive consultations with your medical team, which includes your primary care physician, surgeons, and specialists, are the first step in the procedure.

To develop a customized surgical strategy, your medical history and the particulars of your disease are carefully examined during these consultations.

This entails being aware of the degree of gangrene, the required amputation, and any underlying medical conditions that might affect the treatment.

## Medical Exams And Assessments

You will have several medical examinations and tests performed before the operation to determine your suitability for the procedure and to evaluate your general health. Blood tests for infections, blood sugar, and general organ function are common tests.

To precisely plan the amputation and ascertain the exact spread of the gangrene, imaging tests like CT, MRI, and X-rays are frequently utilized.

 Additionally, if you have a history of heart disease or other cardiovascular issues, a cardiovascular evaluation may be required to make sure your heart can withstand the stress of surgery.

## Instructions & Precautions Before Surgery

To assist you in getting ready for the surgery, your surgeon will provide you with detailed pre-operative instructions. These guidelines frequently call for fasting for a predetermined amount of time before surgery, typically overnight, to guarantee an empty stomach during anesthesia. A few days before the procedure, you might be instructed to cease taking certain drugs, particularly blood thinners, to lower your risk of experiencing severe bleeding. Additionally, to reduce the danger of infection, it's critical to adhere to hygiene recommendations, such as showering with antibacterial soap. Make sure you set up a convenient, easily accessible recuperation area at home and make arrangements for transportation to and from the hospital.

## Psychological Readiness

Getting an amputation can be a very difficult psychological experience. It's critical to discuss any worries or issues you may have regarding the surgery and the ensuing physical changes. It can be helpful to speak with a mental health professional.

They can offer emotional support and coping mechanisms. Speaking with your healthcare team about your worries might also help to allay any confusion and establish reasonable expectations. Peer support groups offer a wonderful platform for meeting people who have experienced similar circumstances and offering reassurance and support.

## Support From Family And Caregivers

Establishing a robust network of support is essential to your recuperation. You should explain the procedure to your family and caregivers, as well as what to anticipate during the healing phase.

They could require assistance with everyday tasks, medicine administration, and emotional support. Involving them in conversations with your medical team might help them better understand your needs and how to

They are the most qualified to help you heal. By getting them ready for potential mental and physical obstacles, you can make sure they'll be able to provide the support that's essential for a quick and complete recovery.

# What To Anticipate On The Surgical Day

You will usually arrive at the hospital or surgical center a few hours before the scheduled procedure on the day of your gangrene amputation surgery.

 After checking in, you'll be brought to the pre-operative area, where you'll make the last-minute preparations and change into a hospital gown. Your vital signs will be taken by a nurse, and you can be given an intravenous (IV) line for medicine and fluids.

The type of anesthetic that will be used during the surgery will be discussed during your meeting with the anesthesiologist. The majority of amputations are carried out while you are unconscious due to a general anesthetic. Regional anesthesia is a medical procedure that can be utilized in some instances to numb the particular location of the body that will be operated on.

You will have a last conversation with your surgeon to go over the specifics of the treatment and to address any last-minute queries or worries before you go to the operating room. The anesthesiologist will place you on the surgery table as soon as you enter the operating room and give you the anesthetic. The amputation will subsequently be carried out by the surgical team, adhering to the meticulously laid out protocols to guarantee a safe and efficient process.

Following the procedure, you'll be brought to a recovery area where medical professionals will keep an eye on your vital signs while you come out of the anesthesia. We'll start pain treatment to keep you comfortable. You might have a drainage tube in place to take out any extra fluid after the surgery, and the surgical site will be bandaged. You will be taken to a hospital room to complete your recuperation under the supervision of the medical staff once you are stable.

# CHAPTER FOUR

## THE SURGICAL METHOD

Gangrene is a dangerous illness in which the tissues die from a lack of blood flow. Amputation is frequently required to stop the disease from spreading further and to save the patient's life.

To stop the infection from spreading and restore functionality, the afflicted tissue is surgically removed during gangrene amputation.

To preserve as much good tissue as possible, the surgeon carefully eliminates the necrotic (dead) tissue throughout the process. This is essential for preserving function and encouraging post-operative recovery.

The amputation procedure may entail the partial or whole removal of the diseased limb or digit, contingent upon the severity of the gangrene.

# Synopsis Of Surgical Procedures

Surgical methods for amputation due to gangrene differ according to the location and extent of the disease. Typical methods include:

Sharp Debridement: In this procedure, the dead tissue is carefully removed using surgical tools like scalpels. It minimizes harm to healthy tissue while enabling precise removal.

Flap procedures: To cover the amputation site and encourage healing, flap procedures may be utilized in situations when significant tissue damage has occurred.

By covering the incision with nearby healthy tissue, flaps lower the risk of infection and promote faster healing.

Closure Techniques: The surgeon uses sutures or staples to close the wound after removing the necrotic tissue.

The objective is to produce a precise, clean closure to hasten healing and avoid complications like infection.

## Methodical Surgical Procedure

Preparation: The surgical team gives the patient anesthesia and makes sure they are positioned correctly. To reduce the chance of infection, they also sterilize the surgical site.

Incision: The gangrene-affected area is incised by the surgeon, who meticulously slices through the skin and surrounding tissues to reveal the necrotic tissue.

Tissue Removal: The surgeon carefully removes the dead tissue with surgical instruments, making sure to preserve healthy tissue for healing and future mobility.

Hemostasis: The surgeon uses cauterizing blood vessels or other hemostatic methods to make sure there is no active bleeding after removing the necrotic tissue.

Closure: Depending on the size and location of the amputation, skin glue, staples, or sutures are used to close the incision.

To encourage the best possible recovery and lower the possibility of problems, the closure is done carefully.

## Pain Management And Anesthesia

To keep the patient relaxed and pain-free throughout the gangrene amputation surgery, anesthesia is essential. Several forms of anesthesia may be utilized, depending on the length of the surgery and the general condition of the patient:

Local anesthetic is frequently applied to individuals who are not suitable candidates for general anesthesia or lesser amputations. It numbs the precise region that is being worked on.

Regional anesthetic: This kind of anesthetic numbs a greater area of the body, such as a whole limb. When amputations are more extensive, it is frequently utilized.

When a patient must be rendered asleep and oblivious to the surgical procedure, general anesthesia is utilized. It guarantees the patient stays still throughout the process and permits total pain management.

## Time Spent During Surgery

The location and severity of the gangrene, the patient's general condition, and the particular surgical technique being employed are some of the variables that might affect how long a gangrene amputation surgery takes.

These procedures often take one to many hours. The total time needed is influenced by elements including the requirement for careful tissue removal and making sure that the closure is done correctly.

## Quick Post-Operative Treatment

The patient's recovery and general health depend heavily on the immediate post-operative treatment following gangrene amputation surgery. Important facets of this care consist of:

Monitoring: The patient is kept under close observation in a recovery area to make sure that all vital signs remain stable and that no serious problems, such as bleeding or infection, arise right away.

Pain Management: Sufficient analgesia is administered to guarantee the patient's comfort. This could involve taking drugs that the surgeon has prescribed orally or intravenously.

Wound Care: To encourage healing and lower the danger of infection, the surgical wound is routinely examined and treated.

The patient and caretakers receive advice on how to properly care for their wounds.

Mobility and Rehabilitation: Early mobility exercises and rehabilitation can help to increase strength and function in the residual limb or get ready for prosthetic fitting, depending on the extent of the amputation.

# CHAPTER FIVE

## AFTER SURGERY RECOVERY

After a gangrene-related amputation, the post-surgical recovery phase is critical and needs close supervision and assistance.

 Patients are thoroughly monitored in a recovery area immediately following the treatment to guarantee stability and appropriate anesthetic reaction.

Keeping an eye on vital signs like blood pressure, oxygen saturation, and heart rate allows medical staff to determine the patient's early state of recovery. Pain management starts as soon as possible to reduce suffering and speed up the healing process.

For a few days, patients usually stay in the hospital to monitor wound healing and make sure there are no issues right away.

Doctors and nurses examine the remaining limb during this period to look for indications of infection or poor circulation. To keep the wound clean and encourage healing, the dressing is changed regularly. Gentle exercises to prevent stiffness and improve circulation in the remaining leg might be started by physical therapists.

Once stable, patients are released from the hospital with comprehensive instructions regarding medication, wound care, and follow-up appointments.

 To reduce complications and maximize healing, patients and caregivers must carefully adhere to these guidelines.

Beginning with physical healing and preparing for possible lifestyle adjustments, this phase signifies the start of adjusting to life after the amputation.

## Techniques For Pain Management

Pain control is essential for those recuperating from an amputation caused by gangrene. Painkillers are given intravenously or orally to manage post-operative pain as soon as surgery is completed. In addition to non-opioid alternatives like acetaminophen or nonsteroidal anti-inflammatory medicines (NSAIDs), these treatments may contain opioids for severe pain.

Pain treatment techniques change as patients heal to address phantom and residual limb pain, which some may endure.

Phantom limb pain is the term for pain or discomfort felt in the absent limb, frequently as a result of the brain misinterpreting nerve impulses.

 Effective management of these symptoms can be achieved with the use of methods like nerve blocks, physical therapy, and psychological interventions like mindfulness and relaxation exercises.

The goal of long-term pain management is to strike a balance between treating pain and reducing drug adverse effects. A mix of prescription drugs, physical therapy, and complementary therapies including transcutaneous electrical nerve stimulation (TENS) or acupuncture may be used to treat this. To modify treatment programs according to each patient's unique pain threshold and response, regular communication with healthcare experts is vital.

## Monitoring And Care For Injuries

After an amputation due to gangrene, wound care is crucial for preventing infections and accelerating healing.

To prevent infection, the surgical wound is covered with a sterile dressing as soon as surgery is completed. To keep the wound dry and clean, the dressing is changed regularly by the healthcare provider's instructions.

Keeping an eye out for infection-related symptoms such as increased redness, edema, or drainage is part of wound monitoring.

Regular wound inspections can help medical professionals monitor the healing process and spot any issues early on. Patients and their carers receive education on how to keep an eye on their wounds at home, including how to spot infection or slow healing and when to call for help.

Sometimes circulation problems or underlying disorders cause wounds to heal more slowly. To encourage healing, advanced wound care methods including negative pressure wound therapy (NPWT) or specialty dressings may be applied. Wound healing is aided by maintaining general health through a balanced diet and adequate hydration.

## Rehabilitation And Physical Therapy

After amputation due to gangrene, physical treatment and rehabilitation are essential for maximizing functional results.

Physical therapists evaluate the patient's residual limb strength and mobility soon after surgery. They create individualized workout plans to enhance balance, joint flexibility, and muscle strength.

Preventing problems like muscular atrophy and joint contractures is the main goal of early rehabilitation. Patients get instructions on how to use mobility aids like crutches and walkers as well as properly transition from bed to a wheelchair.

Therapy gradually moves on to exercises involving standing and walking, if necessary with the aid of prosthetic limbs.

Physical therapy strives to improve independence and quality of life as healing advances. Functional training is a tool that therapists use to mimic everyday tasks like climbing stairs or getting in and out of a car.

To meet their mobility objectives and become proficient with assistive technology users, patients receive continuous guidance and encouragement.

## Adjusting To Assistive Mobility

After an amputation due to gangrene, adapting to mobility aids is a critical part of rehabilitation. Patients can increase their mobility and freedom by using assistive devices including wheelchairs, crutches, walkers, or prosthetic limbs, depending on their needs and the extent of their amputation.

Healthcare practitioners' instruction and training are the first steps in the adaptation process to mobility aids. Patients receive instructions on how to do everyday tasks, navigate various surfaces, and transfer across areas while using the device safely and efficiently. Occupational therapists can help modify living spaces to make room for mobility assistance.

Adaptation for patients utilizing prosthetic limbs entails being familiar with how to use and maintain the device. Patients may begin with simple exercises at first and work their way up to increasingly difficult motions and tasks. Prosthetists recommend routine follow-up sessions to verify the correct fitting of the prosthesis and to make necessary changes for comfort and functionality.

## Mental And Emotional Assistance

Support on both an emotional and psychological level is essential throughout the healing phase following an amputation due to gangrene. Losing a limb can cause a person to feel a variety of feelings, such as sadness, anxiety, and frustration.

Psychologists and counselors are among the healthcare professionals who are vital in resolving emotional difficulties and advancing mental health.

Following surgery, patients receive immediate support from healthcare personnel who address any anxieties or concerns they may have as well as talk about the emotional impact of amputation.

Patients can connect with people who have gone through similar situations through peer support groups or therapy sessions, which offer support and common coping skills.

Ongoing psychological assistance assists patients in adjusting to life without a limb by assisting them in navigating changes in their daily routines, relationships, and self-image.

Relaxation methods and cognitive-behavioral therapy (CBT) can assist control of tension and anxiety associated with adjustment. Patients' resilience and confidence are increased when realistic goals are created and celebrated.

# CHAPTER SIX

## RESURRECTION AS WELL AS PROSTHETICS

The path to rehabilitation and prosthesis use starts after a gangrene amputation. Restoring functionality and adaptability to everyday activities is the goal of this phase.

Following surgery, rehabilitation usually begins soon after with an initial focus on wound healing and pain management for any lingering discomfort. After a patient's health stabilizes, attention turns to getting ready for a prosthetic fitting and mastering the use of the new limb.

Physical therapy is essential to rehabilitation since it helps with strength, flexibility, and coordination. Exercises are customized by therapists to meet each person's unique needs, progressively increasing the endurance and motor skills necessary for using a prosthetic.

To strengthen their limbs and core, patients frequently begin with simple exercises and work their way up to more difficult ones that mimic everyday tasks like walking, climbing stairs, or lifting goods.

Occupational therapy emphasizes everyday chores and functional abilities, which is a supplement to physical treatment. Therapists assist patients in regaining their independence in tasks like grooming, cooking, and maintaining personal hygiene. To ease these chores and guarantee a seamless transition after amputation, they might present adaptive strategies and instruments.

Throughout the rehabilitation process, psychological help is essential for resolving emotional issues and cultivating a positive outlook. Losing a limb requires grieving, accepting oneself, and adjusting to a new body image. Peer support groups and counseling offer a forum for exchanging experiences and problem-solving techniques, fostering mental health in addition to physical healing.

The assessment and fitting of prosthetic devices become more important as rehabilitation advances. Experts evaluate residual limb properties to choose the best prosthetic design. The selection of prosthetic components is influenced by factors such as joint mobility, muscle strength, and skin condition, which ensures maximum comfort and functionality.

## Prosthetics: Types And Applications

Prosthetics have come a long way, with a wide range of designs to suit different requirements and lifestyles. Choosing the best prosthetic option requires an understanding of the types and functionalities:

Transtibial (below-the-knee) prostheses: These are the most popular prostheses, made for people who have had their lower limbs amputated. They usually include a pylon, prosthetic foot, and socket.

Contemporary designs facilitate natural walking patterns by improving stability and energy economy.

Above-Knee (Transfemoral) prostheses: These prostheses have a socket, knee mechanism, pylon, and foot for amputations above the knee. By imitating normal knee movement, advanced knee joints offer stability and control during a variety of activities.

Partial Foot Prosthetics: Specifically made for people who have had part of their foot amputated, these prosthetics improve balance and movement while maintaining the residual foot structure. These may consist of specially designed shoes or insoles to fit particular foot amputations or abnormalities.

Upper Limb Prosthetics: These include sophisticated myoelectric prosthetics that are powered by muscle signals as well as basic cosmetic devices.

They help people regain hand function so they can carry out complex tasks like typing or gripping objects.

Cosmetic prosthetics: These prostheses give a realistic-looking limb to people who are more concerned with looks than functionality.

## Fitting And Personalizing Prosthetic Appearances

Several measures must be taken throughout the painstaking process of prosthetic fitting to guarantee comfort, usefulness, and peak performance:

Initial Assessment: The size, shape, and condition of the residual limb are assessed by a prosthetist. The first choices of prosthetic materials and components are guided by this assessment.

Socket Design: A unique socket is made by the prosthetist to fit snugly over the remaining limb. To maximize socket fit and comfort, cutting-edge methods like computer-aided design (CAD) and 3D printing may be applied.

Component Selection: The prosthetist chooses suitable components, such as knee, foot, and ankle systems, based on the patient's functional goals and lifestyle. Options include both mechanical and microprocessor-driven gadgets, each with special benefits in terms of mobility and stability.

Alignment and Calibration: Balance and natural movement depend on the precise alignment of prosthetic parts. Prosthetists provide optimal performance when walking and other activities by adjusting alignment settings based on gait analysis and patient feedback.

Trial and Adjustment: To test the prosthetic's fit and functionality, patients go through several fitting sessions. Modifications are implemented to optimize comfort, alignment, and general functionality, guaranteeing a perfect prosthetic integration with the body.

## Physiotherapy For The Use Of Prosthetics

To become proficient with prosthetics and achieve functional independence, physical treatment is necessary:

Gait Training: Using the prosthetic limb, therapists work to improve walking gait and balance. Weight shifting, step training, and exercising on different surfaces and inclines are some of the exercises.

Strength and Endurance: Specific workouts improve the strength and endurance of the muscles in the core and residual limb. In the long run, this lessens fatigue and enhances stability when using a prosthetic.

Drills and activities are used by therapists to improve motor control and coordination between the prosthetic limb and the rest of the body. This includes getting practice at things like using stairs, getting around obstructions, and going about daily responsibilities.

Functional Activities: To help patients become used to using their prosthetic limbs in daily duties, therapy sessions mimic real-world settings. Dressing, cooking, and utilizing tools or gadgets are examples of activities.

## Upkeep And Handling Of Prosthetics

The longevity and functionality of prosthetic devices can be extended by appropriate maintenance and care:

Daily Cleaning: Use a mild soap and water solution to clean the prosthetic socket, liner, and other parts regularly to get rid of sweat, debris, and grime.

To avoid fungal infections and skin irritation, completely dry out the area.

Examine the prosthetic regularly for indications of wear, damage, or loose parts. Deal with any problems as soon as possible to avoid pain or possible harm.

Check that the prosthetic socket and liners fit properly. To preserve comfort and functionality, a prosthetist may need to make alterations due to changes in residual limb size or shape.

Component Maintenance: When it comes to maintaining prosthetic knees, ankle systems, and feet, go by the manufacturer's instructions. As advised, lubricate moving parts, and swap out worn-out parts as needed.

Skin Care: To keep the skin of the residual limb healthy, moisturize it every day and try to keep the prosthetic socket from putting too much pressure or friction on it.

# CHAPTER SEVEN

## PERMANENT MAINTENANCE AND MANAGEMENT

After gangrene amputation, there are several important factors to consider to provide the patient with the best possible rehabilitation and quality of life. Preventing problems and promoting the healing process are two main objectives. This usually begins with making sure the surgery site heals appropriately and keeping an eye out for any indications of infection or other problems. It is crucial to take care of wounds properly, which may involve changing dressings regularly, maintaining a clean and dry environment, and adhering to any special instructions given by medical experts.

In long-term care, rehabilitation is also very important. This could entail occupational treatment to help with everyday tasks and physical therapy to help restore strength and mobility. Maximizing independence and functionality despite the amputation is the aim. To increase mobility and offer support, customized orthotics or prosthetics based on the demands and lifestyle of the individual may be advised.

In long-term care, psychological assistance is equally crucial. Emotionally and psychologically, amputation survivors may find it difficult to adjust to life. To assist people deal with the loss, worry, or despair that might come along with such a big transition, counseling or therapy sessions may be helpful. During this period, emotional support from friends, family, and support groups can also be extremely helpful.

Usually, follow-up sessions are arranged with healthcare providers to assess any problems, track the patient's progress, and modify the treatment plan as necessary. By providing continuous support and intervention to encourage healing and general well-being, this continuity of care helps to guarantee that the patient gets what they need.

## Avoiding Issues

Proactive steps to lower infection risk, encourage healing, and preserve general health are necessary to prevent problems following gangrene amputation. Antibiotics may be prescribed right away following surgery to treat or prevent infections.

To reduce the chance of infection, it is essential to maintain a clean, dry surgical site and to adhere to physician advice regarding wound care.

It is crucial to keep an eye out for any indications of complications, such as swelling, redness, increasing discomfort, or drainage from the site.

 It is important to notify medical professionals of any unexpected symptoms as soon as possible so they can evaluate and treat them. When it is feasible, elevating the remaining limb can help with circulation and edema reduction, which will promote recovery.

Reintroducing physical exercise should be done so cautiously and under the supervision of medical professionals.

This increases circulation and lessens the chance of muscular atrophy. An important factor in healing, promoting tissue repair, and general health, is proper nutrition. A well-balanced diet high in protein, vitamins, and minerals helps speed up the healing process and lower the chance of problems.

Sustaining a healthy lifestyle is essential to preventing long-term complications. This includes abstaining from tobacco and excessive alcohol use, both of which can impede healing and circulation.

As long as it's tolerated, regular exercise can enhance general health and cardiovascular health. To avoid problems from chronic illnesses like diabetes or hypertension, it's also critical to manage these conditions.

## Routine Examinations By Doctors

For those who have had gangrene amputations, routine medical checkups are crucial to ensuring their general health and well-being.

During these check-ups, medical professionals usually perform a thorough assessment to monitor the healing process, determine prosthetic needs, and look for any problems.

Healthcare providers may perform physical examinations, go over medical histories, and order diagnostic testing during these visits.

This could entail taking a patient's blood pressure, keeping an eye on their blood sugar levels (particularly if they have diabetes), examining the functioning of their prosthetic device or remaining limb, and analyzing their cardiovascular health.

The frequency of routine examinations can change based on personal circumstances and the particular advice given by medical professionals. Timely intervention and care can greatly influence outcomes and quality of life when complications or difficulties are detected early.

## Modifications To Lifestyle And Good Health

A common adjustment to life after gangrene amputation is changing one's lifestyle to support general health and well-being.

Exercise that is adapted to a person's ability and directed by medical professionals is still vital. Frequent exercise promotes cardiovascular health as well as the preservation of muscle flexibility and strength.

Rehab and continued health are greatly aided by adopting good eating habits. For general health and healing, a balanced diet full of fruits, vegetables, lean proteins, and whole grains offers vital nutrients.

Maintaining a healthy weight through diet supports long-term health objectives and lessens the physical load on the body.

It is highly recommended to stop smoking to increase circulation and lower the chance of problems. Smoking raises the risk of cardiovascular issues and slows the healing process. Reducing alcohol consumption is also recommended because too much alcohol can interfere with prescription drugs and general health.

Adopting a healthy lifestyle also requires emotional well-being. The general quality of life can be enhanced by partaking in hobbies, mindfulness exercises, or support groups—activities that encourage relaxation and stress reduction. Throughout rehabilitation, keeping up social ties with loved ones, friends, and support systems provides emotional support and motivation.

# Resources And Support Groups

For those recuperating from gangrene amputation, support groups and other services are crucial because they offer shared experiences, practical guidance, and emotional support.

These groups could consist of medical experts, community organizations that support amputee care, and peers who have gone through comparable situations.

By joining a support group, people can connect with others going through similar things, exchange coping mechanisms, and get help.

Peer assistance during the healing process might help reduce feelings of loneliness and offer comfort. Topics include prosthetic alternatives, physical rehabilitation exercises, and navigating daily tasks may be discussed in support group meetings.

Apart from support groups, there are other options accessible to help people obtain information and services about the recuperation process after an amputation.

These could include instructional materials, internet discussion boards, workshops, and community resources in your area.

Based on a patient's needs and preferences, healthcare professionals can frequently connect them with appropriate services and suggest reliable sources of information.

## Continuous Medical And Mental Assistance

Following gangrene amputation, ongoing medical and psychological treatment is crucial to long-term management. Physical care entails routinely checking the prosthetic's fit, function, and state of the residual limb. Healthcare professionals look for indications of infection, changes in skin integrity, and problems with using prosthetics.

Sessions of physical therapy may be extended as necessary to maximize balance, strength, and mobility.

Exercises for rehabilitation aid in prosthetic device adaptation, gait mechanic improvement, and general physical function enhancement.

Developing skills for daily tasks is the main goal of occupational therapy, which may also involve instruction in the use of adapted methods or assistive technology.

Providing emotional support continues to be crucial in addressing any psychological issues. Sessions of counseling or therapy offer a secure setting for talking about depression, anxiety, or adjustment issues.

Resilience and emotional well-being can be enhanced by acquiring coping mechanisms and getting emotional support from loved ones, support groups, and healthcare professionals.

Scheduling routine follow-up sessions with healthcare practitioners facilitates continuing evaluation and management of mental and physical health, as well as continuity of care.

After gangrene amputation, this cooperative strategy aids patients in achieving the best possible results, preserving their independence, and improving their general quality of life.

# CHAPTER EIGHT

## CONSIDERING AMPUTATION

Maintaining a fulfilling life while adjusting to new physical realities is a common aspect of living after an amputation. Physical therapy may be necessary in the early stages of amputation adjustment to restore strength and mobility. This technique is essential for learning how to manage everyday duties with fewer limbs or to operate prosthetic devices properly. The transition can be difficult emotionally, requiring time, patience, and support from family, friends, and medical professionals.

One method to make practical improvements in daily life is to learn new techniques for doing routine tasks like cooking, bathing, and dressing. Modifications to the home environment, such as the installation of grab bars in bathrooms or the use of adapted equipment like reachers or dressing aids, may be necessary for these activities. People frequently create routines that include these modifications over time, which promotes increased independence and self-assurance.

Keeping an optimistic outlook is crucial. Many people find that going to counseling or support groups can help them deal with the emotional effects of amputation. Making connections with people who have gone through comparable circumstances can offer support and useful advice for conquering obstacles. Having fun and realistic interests and activities after an amputation can also help people feel normal and well-off.

## Everyday Activities And Life

After an amputation, daily living consists of a combination of new adaptations and known routines. Even simple actions like putting on clothes could be needed for learning new skills or utilizing assistive technology. For example, adaptable clothing with

Velcro or magnetic fasteners makes dressing easier, and elastic shoelaces or Velcro closures can make putting on shoes easier. Stress can be decreased and time can be managed more effectively by arranging daily tasks and making plans in advance.

Sustaining an active lifestyle is essential for general health and well-being. Adaptive sports, cycling, swimming, and other activities can be fun and helpful depending on the degree of amputation and personal ability. Physical therapists frequently offer advice on how to strengthen muscles and improve balance. These improvements can increase mobility and lower the chance of developing secondary health problems.

Planning may be necessary when navigating public areas and transportation. Independence requires accessibility features like elevators, ramps, and reserved parking areas. Wheelchairs and scooters are examples of mobility aids that some people may find useful for longer journeys or uneven terrain. Mobility and freedom can be further enhanced by accessible public transit options or adaptive driving equipment.

## Adaptive Methods And Equipment

After an amputation, adaptive methods and equipment are crucial for managing everyday activities and improving independence.

Depending on the degree of amputation and the intended use, prosthetic devices can range from very basic to quite complex, according to the demands of each individual.

More natural movement and function are made possible by advanced prosthetics, such as hands with sensor technology or knees controlled by microprocessors.

Adaptive equipment and technologies go beyond prosthetics to make certain jobs easier for people to accomplish.

Reachers and grabbers for reaching objects, dressing accessories like zipper pulls or button hooks, and modified kitchen utensils for cooking are a few examples. By regulating lights, appliances, and temperature settings, smart home technology—such as voice-activated assistants or home automation systems—can also make daily tasks easier.

Training and practice are frequently necessary to become a good user of these tools. Occupational therapists are experts in teaching adaptive strategies that are customized to each patient's needs and objectives.

After evaluating functional demands, they suggest the best tools and techniques to increase independence. As people rebuild strength and become accustomed to their prosthetic devices, adaptable procedures and equipment must adjust to meet changing needs. This is ensured by regular evaluations.

# Sustaining Independence

After amputation, maintaining independence necessitates a blend of self-care routines, support networks, and adaptive techniques. Creating a network of family, friends, and medical professionals who can support you is essential for overcoming obstacles and acknowledging your accomplishments. To provide continuous assistance and necessary modifications to prosthetic devices or adaptive equipment, open communication and collaboration with healthcare professionals are essential.

Regular self-care practices enhance independence and general well-being. This entails taking care of any residual limbs to avoid skin problems, eating a balanced diet to aid in healing and energy production, and engaging in regular exercise to build muscle and improve cardiovascular health.

Frequent medical examinations and discussions with experts, such as physical therapists and prosthetists, aid in tracking advancement and quickly addressing any issues.

## Overcoming Emotional And Social Obstacles

Amputation-related social and emotional difficulties must be overcome with self-acceptance, resiliency, and outside help.

Adapting to changes in one's physical attributes and talents can affect confidence and self-worth. Making connections with peers via online communities or support groups offers chances to exchange experiences and coping mechanisms as well as important peer support.

Spreading knowledge about prosthetics and amputations to others aids in encouraging acceptance and understanding in social situations.

Open communication about questions and personal experiences helps debunk myths and promote empathy.

Gaining the ability to be assertive helps people to effectively advocate for their wants and preferences in social situations, the workplace, and public areas.

Motivational Narratives and Accomplishments

People who live with amputations are resilient and determined, as seen by their inspiring experiences and accomplishments.

These narratives frequently highlight people who overcame major obstacles to follow their passions and accomplish personal objectives.

These stories encourage those going through similar experiences, from campaigners raising awareness about limb loss to adapted athletes succeeding in competitive sports.

Success in the arts, careers, rehabilitation, and community service highlight the varied abilities and talents of those who have lost limbs.

These narratives highlight accomplishments of various sizes, showing the potential and opportunities that follow amputation.

They give others hope and motivation to live completely, putting their strengths above their limits and pursuing personal development and fulfillment.

# CHAPTER NINE

## SECONDARY AREAS AND FUTURE GOALS

### Developments In Surgical Methods

Significant improvements have been made in surgical methods for amputations owing to gangrene in recent years. Longer recovery periods and increased risk of problems were common features of traditional treatments.

On the other hand, less invasive treatments like endovascular surgery are becoming more common. These methods decrease blood loss, lessen physical harm to the patient, and shorten hospital stays. To guarantee better results and a quicker recovery for patients, surgeons today employ advanced instruments and methods, such as laser-assisted vascular interventions and precise bone cutting.

The employment of real-time imaging systems during surgery is one noteworthy breakthrough. By using methods such as intraoperative angiography, surgeons can see blood flow and make accurate incisions, protecting as much vital tissue as possible. Furthermore, patient-specific surgical guides are being made via 3D printing technology, which improves amputation accuracy and lowers postoperative complications.

## Advancements In Prosthetics

The state of prosthetic technology has changed dramatically, improving amputees' quality of life significantly. Modern prosthetics are made of lightweight materials that are comfortable and durable, such as carbon fiber. Less physical strain and increased mobility are made possible by these materials. Furthermore, myoelectric prosthetics—which are powered by electrical signals from the user's muscles—have advanced to the point where the artificial limb may be operated more organically and intuitively.

Modern advancements such as osseointegration, in which the prosthetic appendage is fixed to the bone directly, do away with the necessity for socket-based attachments. This technique lowers the chance of skin irritation while providing an increased range of motion and stability. Additionally, users will experience a more smooth and responsive interaction with smart prostheses that are fitted with sensors and microprocessors to adapt to various activities and terrains.

## Investigations And Clinical Trials

Clinical trials and ongoing research are essential to the fight against gangrene and the advancement of amputation techniques. Enhancing early diagnosis and treatment of gangrene is the main goal of studies to avoid the necessity for amputation. Research on stem cell treatment and regenerative medicine, for example, has the potential to lower the incidence of gangrene by repairing injured tissues and restoring blood flow.

The effectiveness of novel drugs and treatment regimens targeted at lowering infection and encouraging quicker healing following amputation is also being investigated in clinical studies. To enhance healing results, novel approaches to wound care, like the use of bioengineered skin grafts and dressings that deliver antibiotics gradually, are being tried. The development of evidence-based procedures that improve patient care and recovery depends on these trials.

## Technology's Place In Rehabilitation

An important part of amputee rehabilitation is technology. Rehabilitation programs are incorporating virtual reality (VR) and augmented reality (AR) to create immersive environments where patients can practice motions and enhance their coordination.

With the help of these technologies, patients can restore their confidence and become used to their prostheses in a secure environment.

Another field where technology is having a big impact is robotics. Wearable technology and robotic exoskeletons support physical therapy by enabling patients to engage in exercises that increase muscle strength and range of motion.

These tools can be customized to meet each person's demands, guaranteeing a unique recovery process. Furthermore, telemedicine technologies provide remote consultations and monitoring, enabling medical professionals to monitor patients' progress and instantly modify treatment programs as needed.

# Future Outlook For Gangrene Treatment And Amputation

The ongoing progress in medical research and technology appears to bode well for the treatment and amputation of gangrene. Driven by advances in genetic and molecular research, personalized medicine is anticipated to have a major impact on improving patient outcomes, lowering the risk of complications, and customizing therapies for specific individuals. Advanced imaging and biomarker analysis are examples of early detection technologies that might facilitate timely intervention and possibly stop gangrene from progressing to the point where amputation is necessary.

More importantly, multidisciplinary approaches that bring together knowledge from disciplines like materials science, robotics, and bioengineering are expected to produce novel solutions for prosthetic design as well as surgical techniques. The precision and effectiveness of patient care will be significantly improved by the incorporation of artificial intelligence (AI) in all aspects, including post-surgical rehabilitation and diagnostics. The prognosis for gangrene and amputation patients will continue to improve with new technology and advancements in research, providing hope for a higher quality of life and greater usefulness.